Birth Log Book

Name:_____

Phone Number:_____

Dates Used:_____

Notes:_____
_____
_____
_____
_____

Date of Birth:	Time of Birth:
Parents' Names:	
Baby Name:	
Parity:	Sex:
Place/Address of Birth:	
Notes/Photo:	

Date of Birth:	Time of Birth:
Parents' Names:	
Baby Name:	
Parity:	Sex:
Place/Address of Birth:	

Notes/Photo:

Date of Birth:	Time of Birth:
Parents' Names:	
Baby Name:	
Parity:	Sex:
Place/Address of Birth:	

Notes/Photo:

Date of Birth:	Time of Birth:
Parents' Names:	
Baby Name:	
Parity:	Sex:
Place/Address of Birth:	

Notes/Photo:

Date of Birth:	Time of Birth:
Parents' Names:	
Baby Name:	
Parity:	Sex:
Place/Address of Birth:	

Notes/Photo:

Date of Birth:	Time of Birth:
Parents' Names:	
Baby Name:	
Parity:	Sex:
Place/Address of Birth:	

Notes/Photo:

Date of Birth:	Time of Birth:
Parents' Names:	
Baby Name:	
Parity:	Sex:
Place/Address of Birth:	
Notes/Photo:	

Date of Birth:	Time of Birth:
Parents' Names:	
Baby Name:	
Parity:	Sex:
Place/Address of Birth:	

Notes/Photo:

Date of Birth:	Time of Birth:
Parents' Names:	
Baby Name:	
Parity:	Sex:
Place/Address of Birth:	
Notes/Photo:	

Date of Birth:	Time of Birth:
Parents' Names:	
Baby Name:	
Parity:	Sex:
Place/Address of Birth:	

Notes/Photo:

Date of Birth:	Time of Birth:
Parents' Names:	
Baby Name:	
Parity:	Sex:
Place/Address of Birth:	

Notes/Photo:

Date of Birth:	Time of Birth:
Parents' Names:	
Baby Name:	
Parity:	Sex:
Place/Address of Birth:	

Notes/Photo:

Date of Birth:	Time of Birth:
Parents' Names:	
Baby Name:	
Parity:	Sex:
Place/Address of Birth:	
Notes/Photo:	

Date of Birth:	Time of Birth:
Parents' Names:	
Baby Name:	
Parity:	Sex:
Place/Address of Birth:	

Notes/Photo:

Date of Birth:	Time of Birth:
Parents' Names:	
Baby Name:	
Parity:	Sex:
Place/Address of Birth:	

Notes/Photo:

Date of Birth:	Time of Birth:
Parents' Names:	
Baby Name:	
Parity:	Sex:
Place/Address of Birth:	

Notes/Photo:

Date of Birth:	Time of Birth:
Parents' Names:	
Baby Name:	
Parity:	Sex:
Place/Address of Birth:	
Notes/Photo:	

Date of Birth:	Time of Birth:

Parents' Names:

Baby Name:

Parity:	Sex:

Place/Address of Birth:

Notes/Photo:

Date of Birth:	Time of Birth:
Parents' Names:	
Baby Name:	
Parity:	Sex:
Place/Address of Birth:	
Notes/Photo:	

Date of Birth:	Time of Birth:

Parents' Names:

Baby Name:

Parity:	Sex:

Place/Address of Birth:

Notes/Photo:

Date of Birth:	Time of Birth:
Parents' Names:	
Baby Name:	
Parity:	Sex:
Place/Address of Birth:	

Notes/Photo:

Date of Birth:	Time of Birth:
Parents' Names:	
Baby Name:	
Parity:	Sex:
Place/Address of Birth:	

Notes/Photo:

Date of Birth:	Time of Birth:
Parents' Names:	
Baby Name:	
Parity:	Sex:
Place/Address of Birth:	
Notes/Photo:	

Date of Birth:	Time of Birth:
Parents' Names:	
Baby Name:	
Parity:	Sex:
Place/Address of Birth:	

Notes/Photo:

Date of Birth:	Time of Birth:

Parents' Names:

Baby Name:

Parity:	Sex:

Place/Address of Birth:

Notes/Photo:

Date of Birth:	Time of Birth:
Parents' Names:	
Baby Name:	
Parity:	Sex:
Place/Address of Birth:	

Notes/Photo:

Date of Birth:	Time of Birth:
Parents' Names:	
Baby Name:	
Parity:	Sex:
Place/Address of Birth:	

Notes/Photo:

Date of Birth:	Time of Birth:
Parents' Names:	
Baby Name:	
Parity:	Sex:
Place/Address of Birth:	

Notes/Photo:

Date of Birth:	Time of Birth:
Parents' Names:	
Baby Name:	
Parity:	Sex:
Place/Address of Birth:	
Notes/Photo:	

Date of Birth:	Time of Birth:
Parents' Names:	
Baby Name:	
Parity:	Sex:
Place/Address of Birth:	

Notes/Photo:

Date of Birth:	Time of Birth:
Parents' Names:	
Baby Name:	
Parity:	Sex:
Place/Address of Birth:	

Notes/Photo:

Date of Birth:	Time of Birth:
Parents' Names:	
Baby Name:	
Parity:	Sex:
Place/Address of Birth:	

Notes/Photo:

Date of Birth:	Time of Birth:
Parents' Names:	
Baby Name:	
Parity:	Sex:
Place/Address of Birth:	
Notes/Photo:	

Date of Birth:	Time of Birth:
Parents' Names:	
Baby Name:	
Parity:	Sex:
Place/Address of Birth:	

Notes/Photo:

Date of Birth:	Time of Birth:
Parents' Names:	
Baby Name:	
Parity:	Sex:
Place/Address of Birth:	
Notes/Photo:	

Date of Birth:	Time of Birth:

Parents' Names:

Baby Name:

Parity:	Sex:

Place/Address of Birth:

Notes/Photo:

Date of Birth:	Time of Birth:
Parents' Names:	
Baby Name:	
Parity:	Sex:
Place/Address of Birth:	

Notes/Photo:

Date of Birth:	Time of Birth:
Parents' Names:	

Baby Name:

Parity:	Sex:

Place/Address of Birth:

Notes/Photo:

Date of Birth:	Time of Birth:
Parents' Names:	
Baby Name:	
Parity:	Sex:
Place/Address of Birth:	

Notes/Photo:

Date of Birth:	Time of Birth:
Parents' Names:	
Baby Name:	
Parity:	Sex:
Place/Address of Birth:	
Notes/Photo:	

Date of Birth:	Time of Birth:
Parents' Names:	
Baby Name:	
Parity:	Sex:
Place/Address of Birth:	

Notes/Photo:

Date of Birth:	Time of Birth:

Parents' Names:

Baby Name:

Parity:	Sex:

Place/Address of Birth:

Notes/Photo:

Date of Birth:	Time of Birth:
Parents' Names:	
Baby Name:	
Parity:	Sex:
Place/Address of Birth:	

Notes/Photo:

Date of Birth:	Time of Birth:
Parents' Names:	
Baby Name:	
Parity:	Sex:
Place/Address of Birth:	

Notes/Photo:

Date of Birth:	Time of Birth:
Parents' Names:	
Baby Name:	
Parity:	Sex:
Place/Address of Birth:	

Notes/Photo:

Date of Birth:	Time of Birth:
Parents' Names:	

Baby Name:	
Parity:	Sex:
Place/Address of Birth:	

Notes/Photo:

Date of Birth:	Time of Birth:
Parents' Names:	
Baby Name:	
Parity:	Sex:
Place/Address of Birth:	

Notes/Photo:

Date of Birth:	Time of Birth:

Parents' Names:

Baby Name:

Parity:	Sex:

Place/Address of Birth:

Notes/Photo:

Date of Birth:	Time of Birth:
Parents' Names:	
Baby Name:	
Parity:	Sex:
Place/Address of Birth:	

Notes/Photo:

Date of Birth:	Time of Birth:

Parents' Names:

Baby Name:

Parity:	Sex:

Place/Address of Birth:

Notes/Photo:

Date of Birth:	Time of Birth:
Parents' Names:	
Baby Name:	
Parity:	Sex:
Place/Address of Birth:	

Notes/Photo:

Date of Birth:	Time of Birth:
Parents' Names:	
Baby Name:	
Parity:	Sex:
Place/Address of Birth:	

Notes/Photo:

Date of Birth:	Time of Birth:

Parents' Names:

Baby Name:

Parity:	Sex:

Place/Address of Birth:

Notes/Photo:

Date of Birth:	Time of Birth:
Parents' Names:	

Baby Name:	
Parity:	Sex:
Place/Address of Birth:	

Notes/Photo:

Date of Birth:	Time of Birth:

Parents' Names:

Baby Name:

Parity:	Sex:

Place/Address of Birth:

Notes/Photo:

Date of Birth:	Time of Birth:
Parents' Names:	
Baby Name:	
Parity:	Sex:
Place/Address of Birth:	

Notes/Photo:

Date of Birth:	Time of Birth:

Parents' Names:

Baby Name:

Parity:	Sex:

Place/Address of Birth:

Notes/Photo:

Date of Birth:	Time of Birth:
Parents' Names:	
Baby Name:	
Parity:	Sex:
Place/Address of Birth:	

Notes/Photo:

Date of Birth:	Time of Birth:
Parents' Names:	
Baby Name:	
Parity:	Sex:
Place/Address of Birth:	

Notes/Photo:

Date of Birth:	Time of Birth:
Parents' Names:	
Baby Name:	
Parity:	Sex:
Place/Address of Birth:	

Notes/Photo:

Date of Birth:	Time of Birth:
Parents' Names:	
Baby Name:	
Parity:	Sex:
Place/Address of Birth:	
Notes/Photo:	

Date of Birth:	Time of Birth:
Parents' Names:	
Baby Name:	
Parity:	Sex:
Place/Address of Birth:	

Notes/Photo:

Date of Birth:	Time of Birth:
Parents' Names:	
Baby Name:	
Parity:	Sex:
Place/Address of Birth:	

Notes/Photo:

Date of Birth:	Time of Birth:
Parents' Names:	
Baby Name:	
Parity:	Sex:
Place/Address of Birth:	

Notes/Photo:

Date of Birth:	Time of Birth:
Parents' Names:	
Baby Name:	
Parity:	Sex:
Place/Address of Birth:	

Notes/Photo:

Date of Birth:	Time of Birth:
Parents' Names:	
Baby Name:	
Parity:	Sex:
Place/Address of Birth:	

Notes/Photo:

Date of Birth:	Time of Birth:
Parents' Names:	
Baby Name:	
Parity:	Sex:
Place/Address of Birth:	

Notes/Photo:

Date of Birth:	Time of Birth:
Parents' Names:	
Baby Name:	
Parity:	Sex:
Place/Address of Birth:	

Notes/Photo:

Date of Birth:	Time of Birth:
Parents' Names:	
Baby Name:	
Parity:	Sex:
Place/Address of Birth:	

Notes/Photo:

Date of Birth:	Time of Birth:
Parents' Names:	
Baby Name:	
Parity:	Sex:
Place/Address of Birth:	

Notes/Photo:

Date of Birth:	Time of Birth:
Parents' Names:	
Baby Name:	
Parity:	Sex:
Place/Address of Birth:	

Notes/Photo:

Date of Birth:	Time of Birth:
Parents' Names:	
Baby Name:	
Parity:	Sex:
Place/Address of Birth:	

Notes/Photo:

Date of Birth:	Time of Birth:
Parents' Names:	
Baby Name:	
Parity:	Sex:
Place/Address of Birth:	

Notes/Photo:

Date of Birth:	Time of Birth:
Parents' Names:	
Baby Name:	
Parity:	Sex:
Place/Address of Birth:	

Notes/Photo:

Date of Birth:	Time of Birth:
Parents' Names:	
Baby Name:	
Parity:	Sex:
Place/Address of Birth:	

Notes/Photo:

Date of Birth:	Time of Birth:
Parents' Names:	

Baby Name:	
Parity:	Sex:

Place/Address of Birth:

Notes/Photo:

Date of Birth:	Time of Birth:
Parents' Names:	
Baby Name:	
Parity:	Sex:
Place/Address of Birth:	

Notes/Photo:

Date of Birth:	Time of Birth:
Parents' Names:	
Baby Name:	
Parity:	Sex:
Place/Address of Birth:	

Notes/Photo:

Date of Birth:	Time of Birth:
Parents' Names:	
Baby Name:	
Parity:	Sex:
Place/Address of Birth:	

Notes/Photo:

Date of Birth:	Time of Birth:
Parents' Names:	
Baby Name:	
Parity:	Sex:
Place/Address of Birth:	

Notes/Photo:

Date of Birth:	Time of Birth:

Parents' Names:

Baby Name:

Parity:	Sex:

Place/Address of Birth:

Notes/Photo:

Date of Birth:	Time of Birth:
Parents' Names:	
Baby Name:	
Parity:	Sex:
Place/Address of Birth:	
Notes/Photo:	

Date of Birth:	Time of Birth:
Parents' Names:	
Baby Name:	
Parity:	Sex:
Place/Address of Birth:	

Notes/Photo:

Date of Birth:	Time of Birth:
Parents' Names:	
Baby Name:	
Parity:	Sex:
Place/Address of Birth:	

Notes/Photo:

Date of Birth:	Time of Birth:
Parents' Names:	
Baby Name:	
Parity:	Sex:
Place/Address of Birth:	

Notes/Photo:

Date of Birth:	Time of Birth:
Parents' Names:	

Baby Name:	
Parity:	Sex:
Place/Address of Birth:	

Notes/Photo:

Date of Birth:	Time of Birth:
Parents' Names:	
Baby Name:	
Parity:	Sex:
Place/Address of Birth:	

Notes/Photo:

Date of Birth:	Time of Birth:
Parents' Names:	
Baby Name:	
Parity:	Sex:
Place/Address of Birth:	

Notes/Photo:

Date of Birth:	Time of Birth:
Parents' Names:	
Baby Name:	
Parity:	Sex:
Place/Address of Birth:	

Notes/Photo:

Date of Birth:	Time of Birth:
Parents' Names:	
Baby Name:	
Parity:	Sex:
Place/Address of Birth:	

Notes/Photo:

Date of Birth:	Time of Birth:
Parents' Names:	
Baby Name:	
Parity:	Sex:
Place/Address of Birth:	
Notes/Photo:	

Date of Birth:	Time of Birth:
Parents' Names:	
Baby Name:	
Parity:	Sex:
Place/Address of Birth:	

Notes/Photo:

Date of Birth:	Time of Birth:
Parents' Names:	
Baby Name:	
Parity:	Sex:
Place/Address of Birth:	

Notes/Photo:

Date of Birth:	Time of Birth:
Parents' Names:	
Baby Name:	
Parity:	Sex:
Place/Address of Birth:	

Notes/Photo:

Date of Birth:	Time of Birth:
Parents' Names:	
Baby Name:	
Parity:	Sex:
Place/Address of Birth:	
Notes/Photo:	

Date of Birth:	Time of Birth:
Parents' Names:	
Baby Name:	
Parity:	Sex:
Place/Address of Birth:	

Notes/Photo:

Date of Birth:	Time of Birth:
Parents' Names:	
Baby Name:	
Parity:	Sex:
Place/Address of Birth:	

Notes/Photo:

Date of Birth:	Time of Birth:
Parents' Names:	
Baby Name:	
Parity:	Sex:
Place/Address of Birth:	

Notes/Photo:

Date of Birth:	Time of Birth:
Parents' Names:	
Baby Name:	
Parity:	Sex:
Place/Address of Birth:	

Notes/Photo:

Date of Birth:	Time of Birth:
Parents' Names:	
Baby Name:	
Parity:	Sex:
Place/Address of Birth:	

Notes/Photo:

Date of Birth:	Time of Birth:
Parents' Names:	
Baby Name:	
Parity:	Sex:
Place/Address of Birth:	

Notes/Photo:

Date of Birth:	Time of Birth:
Parents' Names:	
Baby Name:	
Parity:	Sex:
Place/Address of Birth:	

Notes/Photo:

Date of Birth:	Time of Birth:
Parents' Names:	
Baby Name:	
Parity:	Sex:
Place/Address of Birth:	

Notes/Photo:

Date of Birth:	Time of Birth:
Parents' Names:	
Baby Name:	
Parity:	Sex:
Place/Address of Birth:	

Notes/Photo:

Date of Birth:	Time of Birth:
Parents' Names:	
Baby Name:	
Parity:	Sex:
Place/Address of Birth:	

Notes/Photo:

Date of Birth:	Time of Birth:
Parents' Names:	
Baby Name:	
Parity:	Sex:
Place/Address of Birth:	

Notes/Photo:

Date of Birth:	Time of Birth:
Parents' Names:	
Baby Name:	
Parity:	Sex:
Place/Address of Birth:	

Notes/Photo:

Date of Birth:	Time of Birth:
Parents' Names:	
Baby Name:	
Parity:	Sex:
Place/Address of Birth:	

Notes/Photo:

Date of Birth:	Time of Birth:
Parents' Names:	
Baby Name:	
Parity:	Sex:
Place/Address of Birth:	

Notes/Photo:

Date of Birth:	Time of Birth:
Parents' Names:	
Baby Name:	
Parity:	Sex:
Place/Address of Birth:	

Notes/Photo:

Date of Birth:	Time of Birth:
Parents' Names:	
Baby Name:	
Parity:	Sex:
Place/Address of Birth:	

Notes/Photo:

Date of Birth:	Time of Birth:
Parents' Names:	
Baby Name:	
Parity:	Sex:
Place/Address of Birth:	

Notes/Photo:

Date of Birth:	Time of Birth:
Parents' Names:	
Baby Name:	
Parity:	Sex:
Place/Address of Birth:	

Notes/Photo:

Date of Birth:	Time of Birth:
Parents' Names:	
Baby Name:	
Parity:	Sex:
Place/Address of Birth:	

Notes/Photo:

Date of Birth:	Time of Birth:
Parents' Names:	
Baby Name:	
Parity:	Sex:
Place/Address of Birth:	
Notes/Photo:	

Date of Birth:	Time of Birth:
Parents' Names:	
Baby Name:	
Parity:	Sex:
Place/Address of Birth:	

Notes/Photo:

Date of Birth:	Time of Birth:
Parents' Names:	
Baby Name:	
Parity:	Sex:
Place/Address of Birth:	

Notes/Photo:

Date of Birth:	Time of Birth:
Parents' Names:	
Baby Name:	
Parity:	Sex:
Place/Address of Birth:	

Notes/Photo:

Date of Birth:	Time of Birth:
Parents' Names:	
Baby Name:	
Parity:	Sex:
Place/Address of Birth:	

Notes/Photo:

Manufactured by Amazon.ca
Bolton, ON